Chair Yoga for Seniors Made Easy:

Quick and Simple Exercises for Ages 60+, Men Over 40, and a Path to Weight Loss.

+

BONUS

Anne Herzog

Copyright © 2024 by Anne Herzog

About the Author

Anne Herzog is a distinguished yoga instructor whose journey into the world of yoga spans over 25 years. Originally from Switzerland, Anne has spent much of her life immersed in the rich and transformative practice of yoga in India. Her deep connection to the practice and her extensive experience have made her a respected figure in the yoga community.

Throughout her career, Anne has traveled to over 10 countries, enriching her understanding of yoga and its diverse practices. Her global experiences have provided her with a unique perspective on the universal benefits of yoga, which she seamlessly integrates into her teachings. Anne's approach to yoga is deeply rooted in her personal journey of growth and discovery. She is dedicated to helping others find balance, strength, and tranquility through their own yoga practice. Her passion for yoga is matched only by her love for her family. Anne is happily married and a devoted mother to three beautiful children. Her family continues to be a source of inspiration and support as she shares her knowledge and passion for yoga with the world. Anne Herzog's dedication to yoga and her rich cultural experiences bring a profound depth to her teaching, making her a cherished guide for those seeking to enhance their well-being through this ancient practice.

Table of Contents

Introduction

Welcome to **Chair Yoga for Seniors Made Easy!** Whether you're a beginner or have years of yoga experience, this book is crafted to introduce you to the accessible and enriching practice of chair yoga, specifically designed for seniors. As we grow older, preserving both physical and mental health becomes increasingly essential. Chair yoga offers a gentle yet effective way to maintain flexibility, strength, and balance, all while practicing in the comfort of a chair. It combines physical movement with relaxation techniques, making it ideal for those who may find traditional yoga postures more challenging.

In this book, you'll discover everything you need to start or deepen your chair yoga practice. We begin with the basics, covering the origins of chair yoga and why it's particularly beneficial for seniors. You'll learn how to create your practice space, choose the right chair, and prepare your body for movement. Each chapter presents a variety of chair yoga poses, complete with step-by-step instructions and adjustments to accommodate different levels of ability. You'll find sample routines to follow, as well as guidance on developing your own personalized practice. We also address common concerns such as joint health, back pain relief, improved circulation, and enhanced balance, offering targeted poses to meet these needs.

But chair yoga is more than just physical exercise—it also incorporates mindfulness and relaxation techniques to reduce stress, enhance mental clarity, and promote overall well-being. Throughout this book, we will guide you in incorporating these elements into your daily life, helping you fully experience the benefits of chair yoga. This practice is not merely about staying active; it's about embracing a lifestyle that fosters health, happiness, and community. As you explore these pages, I encourage you to approach chair yoga with an open mind and heart. Together, we will discover how this practice can enhance your life, bringing greater ease and joy to your everyday routine.

Let your journey of chair yoga begin—welcome!

Understanding Chair Yoga

What is Chair Yoga?

Chair yoga is a gentle form of yoga in which postures are performed while seated or with the support of a chair. It is particularly suited for individuals with physical limitations, including seniors or those who find traditional yoga sessions too demanding. This practice is also ideal for beginners or anyone seeking a more gentle approach to yoga.

As a modified version of traditional yoga, chair yoga allows for poses to be practiced from a seated position. It typically incorporates gentle stretches, breathing exercises, and meditation techniques. Unlike standard yoga, which often involves standing or balancing poses on a mat, chair yoga is highly adaptable. Whether you are recovering from an injury, needing a short break at your desk, or feeling low on energy, chair yoga offers a simple yet effective way to reset.

Elements of chair yoga can even be integrated into a traditional Hatha yoga class, particularly for those with balance challenges or difficulty transitioning between floor poses. Rooted in traditional yoga—an ancient practice with over 5,000 years of history—many classical yoga postures can be adapted for a seated position or modified with the aid of a chair. This makes chair yoga an accessible and enjoyable practice for individuals of all experience levels, including seniors.

Comparison With Traditional Yoga

If you're a yoga enthusiast looking to start your practice, you may be wondering: how do I choose between chair yoga and traditional yoga classes? Don't worry—this book is here to help guide your decision. Yoga comes in many styles and forms, each offering unique benefits for both body and mind. Two popular options are traditional yoga and chair yoga. By the time you finish this book, you'll have a clear understanding of both, enabling you to choose the style that best suits your abilities and preferences. Let's dive in!

The word "yoga" means union, symbolizing the connection of the physical, mental, and spiritual self. When practiced regularly, yoga allows you to gain control over both your body and mind. Now, you might be asking yourself: can chair yoga offer the same benefits as traditional yoga? Move on with me.....

Finding the Right Fit

Finding the right yoga style becomes much easier once you know the transformation you're aiming for. While you may not turn into Spiderman or Superman, yoga—whether traditional or chair-based—can help you achieve flexibility and mindfulness. However, both styles have their limitations, which should be considered before making your choice. Let's explore the pros and cons of traditional yoga and chair yoga to guide your decision.

Traditional Yoga

Traditional yoga involves the full engagement of various body parts in a series of physical postures. However, its focus extends beyond physical movement, emphasizing the mind-body connection through controlled breathing techniques and spiritual awareness.

Pros:

1. Holistic Health Benefits

Traditional yoga offers a comprehensive approach to well-being. It goes beyond physical postures, integrating mental and spiritual aspects. This practice encompasses Asana (physical postures), Pranayama (breathing exercises), Yama (self-discipline), and Niyama (guiding principles for life), providing a holistic path to health.

2. Strength and Flexibility

Many traditional yoga postures are weight-bearing, requiring no external props like chairs. As a result, practitioners engage and strengthen muscles and joints, ultimately maximizing both strength and flexibility.

3. Stress Reduction

Traditional yoga places great emphasis on breath control, fostering balance in internal energy. This focus on Pranayama has a profound impact on reducing stress and calming the mind by influencing stress hormones.

Cons:

1. Physical Demands

While traditional yoga offers numerous health benefits, certain styles can be physically demanding, requiring a degree of fitness and flexibility that may be challenging for beginners or individuals with physical limitations.

2. Learning Curve and Mental Frustration

Though yoga is designed to promote relaxation and health, some traditional poses can be complex. For beginners, the learning process can be difficult, and without proper guidance, frustration or even injury may occur.

Ultimately, the choice between chair yoga and traditional yoga depends on your current physical condition, fitness level, and experience. If you're looking for a gentle, accessible practice, chair yoga may be the ideal option. On the other hand, if you're seeking a more comprehensive, holistic approach, traditional yoga might be the perfect fit.

Chair Yoga

Chair yoga was developed with adaptability in mind, making it accessible to those with limited flexibility. Despite being a more gentle practice, chair yoga still emphasizes breathing techniques, mindfulness, and relaxation, fostering a deep mind-body connection, just like traditional yoga.

Pros:

1. Accessibility

Chair yoga is an excellent choice for individuals with limited mobility, seniors, or those recovering from injuries. The use of a chair provides a stable foundation, making the practice accessible to a wider range of participants.

2. Adaptability

This form of yoga is highly adaptable, allowing for modifications in postures to accommodate different physical abilities. Whether you're new to yoga or a seasoned practitioner, chair yoga can offer a customized, comfortable, yet challenging experience that enhances both mind and body.

3. Joint-Friendly

Chair yoga is ideal for those with arthritis or joint issues, as it promotes joint flexibility, strength, and balance without putting strain on the joints. The support of a chair enables you to flow through gentle movements, leaving you feeling relaxed and refreshed.

4. Inclusive Community

Chair yoga fosters an inclusive environment where people of all fitness levels and physical conditions can practice together. It offers a supportive, non-intimidating space, making it a wonderful way to connect with others and boost overall well-being.

Cons:

1. Limited Intensity

Chair yoga may not provide the same high-intensity, heart-pumping workout that you might experience with traditional yoga.

2. Restricted Range of Poses

Due to the reliance on a chair for support, certain poses may not be possible, potentially limiting the variety and excitement of the practice.

Choosing Between Chair Yoga and Traditional Yoga

When deciding between chair yoga and traditional yoga, the first step is to assess yourself. Consider which type of yoga best suits your physical abilities, health conditions, personal preferences, and goals. Use the following guideline to help make your decision.

Is it Suitable for All Physical Abilities?

If you have limited mobility, balance challenges, or difficulty getting up and down from the floor, chair yoga may be the ideal choice. It offers a supportive practice that accommodates a range of physical abilities. On the other hand, if you're seeking a more physically demanding experience and possess greater flexibility and fitness, traditional yoga may be more appropriate. Traditional yoga includes standing, balancing, and floor-based postures.

Is it Adaptable to Health Conditions?

Your health condition can greatly influence your choice of yoga style. Chair yoga is particularly well-suited for individuals managing chronic conditions, injuries, or health concerns such as arthritis, back pain, or joint issues. However, traditional yoga can also be adapted to meet your needs if you're generally healthy but face certain limitations. In either case, it's essential to consult with a healthcare professional or an experienced yoga instructor before starting, especially if you have specific health concerns.

Do Personal Preferences and Goals Matter?

Absolutely. Personal preferences and goals play a key role in your decision. If you prefer a more relaxed and gentle practice that balances flexibility and mindfulness, chair yoga may be the better fit. If you're looking for a more dynamic practice that includes balancing and challenging postures, traditional yoga could be the right choice. Regardless of which style you choose, yoga will bring positivity and joy to your life. Ready to explore the poses you can practice with both styles? Read on!

Chair Yoga Adaptations vs. Classic Yoga Poses

What postures and practices are included in chair yoga and traditional yoga? If you're still uncertain about what to expect from these yoga styles, here's a brief overview of the adaptations in chair yoga and the traditional practices found in classic yoga.

Chair Yoga Poses
Grab a chair and try these to begin your practice!
- Seated Poses
  Chair yoga primarily focuses on seated postures that involve stretching, flexing, and relaxing. Poses like neck stretches, seated twists, and forward bends are common in this practice.
- Chair-Assisted Standing Poses
  A chair can be used for support when performing standing poses, which help to strengthen your legs.
- Breathing Exercises
  Sitting in a chair provides comfort and relaxation, making it an ideal setting for practicing breathing awareness and controlled breathing techniques.
- Adaptations and Use of Props
  Chair yoga is highly adaptable, allowing for the use of props such as blocks, cushions, or pillows to enhance

comfort and support. The goal is to experience the benefits of yoga while maintaining comfort.

Traditional Yoga Practices

In contrast, traditional or classic yoga places greater emphasis on precision and mastery of postures and breathwork, creating a harmonious connection between the body and mind. Here are some of the key traditional yoga practices:

- Hatha Yoga
  Hatha yoga focuses on foundational postures and breath control, making it an excellent choice for beginners.
- Vinyasa Yoga
  Vinyasa yoga features continuous, flowing sequences synchronized with breath, offering dynamic energy and movement.
- Ashtanga Yoga
  Ashtanga yoga emphasizes discipline and structure, following a set sequence of postures.
- Iyengar Yoga
  A modified form of classic yoga, Iyengar yoga prioritizes precision and alignment, often using props for support. This practice is ideal for those seeking therapeutic benefits.
- Kundalini Yoga
  Kundalini yoga centers on breathwork to release tension and unlock dormant energy, providing a spiritual and transformative experience.

Which Yoga Style is Right for You?

Deciding between chair yoga and traditional yoga can be challenging, but understanding their differences will help you make an informed choice. Remember, yoga isn't solely about perfecting postures—it's also about restoring your body's energy through mindful movements and breathwork. Ultimately, the most important factor is the effort you dedicate to your practice. Choose the style that resonates with you, and enjoy the transformative benefits of a regular yoga routine!

Who can practice chair yoga?

It is often misunderstood that chair yoga is solely for seniors or individuals recovering from injuries, but this is far from true. In fact, chair yoga can benefit busy parents, office workers, frequent travelers, and even students. Given the sedentary nature of modern life, chair yoga is an ideal solution to counteract the negative effects of prolonged sitting. Rather than focusing on challenging poses, this practice prioritizes comfort and ease.

Why Choose Chair Yoga?

Top Ten Benefits of Chair Yoga

1. Enhancing Accessibility

Traditional yoga often involves transitioning from standing to the floor, which may be challenging for those with mobility issues, disabilities, or injuries. Chair yoga modifies postures, making them accessible to a wider audience. As long as you can sit in a chair, you can practice chair yoga. This approach is also well-suited for workplace environments, where space or clothing changes might be limited.

2. Promoting an Active Lifestyle

With sedentary lifestyles becoming more common, it's important to incorporate physical activity into daily routines. National health guidelines encourage regular movement throughout the day, and chair yoga is an excellent way to add brief, effective stretches between long periods of sitting.

3. Relieving Tension and Pain

Extended sitting often leads to poor posture, causing tension in the back, neck, and shoulders. Chair yoga helps release these physical stresses by improving mobility and strength. Studies have shown that regular yoga practice can alleviate pain, including lower back, shoulder, and neck discomfort, while enhancing posture awareness over time.

4. Improving Sleep Quality

Light physical exercise, such as chair yoga, has been shown to improve sleep quality. Engaging in a chair yoga routine can help you unwind after a busy day, reducing stress and leading to better rest and increased energy levels.

5. Increasing Flexibility

Flexibility tends to decrease with age, and prolonged sitting or repetitive movements can accelerate stiffness. Yoga has been proven to safely increase flexibility, strength, and balance, helping you maintain mobility as you age. Regular practice over time can lead to significant improvements in flexibility and range of motion.

6. Building Strength and Stability

Adults are advised to engage in strength-building activities at least twice a week to maintain healthy muscles, bones, and joints. Chair yoga exercises, which use bodyweight resistance, can help enhance muscle strength and stability, providing an excellent starting point for those new to strength training.

7. Improving Balance and Preventing Falls

Good balance is essential for preventing accidents and injuries, especially later in life. Chair yoga allows for safe, controlled balance exercises that engage core and leg muscles. Practicing these movements regularly can help train your body to respond more effectively to unexpected changes in position, improving balance over time.

8. Reducing Stress

Chair yoga provides an opportunity to focus on your breath and body, which helps calm the mind and reduce stress levels. Research has shown that physical activities like yoga can improve mental well-being by lowering anxiety, depression, and stress, while enhancing self-esteem and cognitive function.

9. Boosting Energy Levels

Throughout a busy day, energy levels can naturally decline, leading to reduced productivity. Incorporating short chair yoga breaks into your routine can help restore energy, increase focus, and improve overall efficiency. With no need for special equipment or clothing, chair yoga is a convenient way to recharge.

10. Fostering Social Connections

Learning new skills, such as chair yoga, can provide opportunities for personal growth and confidence building. Practicing in a group setting, whether at work or in the community, encourages social bonding and the development of soft and social skills, fostering a sense of connection and belonging.

Common Risks and Safe Practices in Chair Yoga

While chair yoga is generally considered a low-risk activity, there are a few safety precautions to keep in mind to ensure a safe and effective practice. Potential risks such as slipping, overstretching, or incorrect posture can be mitigated by following these guidelines:

- Use a sturdy, non-wheeled chair to prevent slipping or instability.
- Move slowly and carefully to avoid overstretching or injury.
- Pay attention to your body's signals to avoid pushing yourself too hard.

- Check your alignment during poses to maximize benefits and reduce the risk of injury.

Creating an Optimal Chair Yoga Environment

Setting up a suitable space for chair yoga can enhance your overall experience and promote better outcomes. Even if you are attending a session with a yoga therapist, you can request adjustments to the environment. Consider the following:

- Ensure the area is calm, comfortable, and free of clutter.
- Allow ample space for movement and stretching.
- Use a sturdy, non-wheeled chair with a firm seat and back support.
- Place a yoga mat or non-slip rug under your feet for added stability.
- Ensure the space is well-lit for better visibility.
- Add personal touches, such as cushions, candles, or photos, to create a relaxing atmosphere.
- If necessary, have someone nearby to assist or supervise.

Choosing the Right Clothing for Chair Yoga

Wearing appropriate attire can enhance comfort and range of motion during chair yoga. Opt for clothing that is both comfortable and functional:

- Choose stretchy, breathable fabrics that allow for full movement.

- Loose-fitting tops and pants or leggings are ideal for promoting ease of movement and circulation.
- Avoid overly baggy clothing, as it may interfere with poses or get caught on the chair during movement.

Chair Yoga Exercises for Seniors

As a yoga therapist, I understand that achieving optimal results for specific goals requires yoga practices tailored to the individual. A one-size-fits-all approach won't address unique concerns such as back pain or anxiety. However, to provide a general idea of what chair yoga exercises for seniors might look like, here are six examples:

1. Seated Mountain Pose
This foundational pose helps promote proper posture and strengthens the spine. It can also alleviate back pain. While seated, place your feet flat on the ground, elongate your spine on an inhale, and release any tension as you exhale.

2. Gentle Seated Twist
Twists are beneficial for digestion, spinal flexibility, and easing back pain. To perform, sit upright with your feet on the floor, lengthen your spine, and gently twist at the hips to one side, then switch.

3. Chair Warrior Poses

Both Chair Warrior I and II can be adapted for seated practice to strengthen muscles, improve balance, and enhance stability. For Warrior I, sit sideways, bend one leg at a 90-degree angle, extend the other behind you, and raise your arms toward the ceiling. For Warrior II, extend your arms parallel to the ground while sitting sideways and looking over your bent knee.

4. Chair Pigeon Pose

This forward fold stretches muscles in the lower back, hips, and hamstrings, improving flexibility. To practice, keep one foot on the floor, cross the other leg so its ankle rests over the opposite knee, and gently fold forward from the hips.

5. Seated Diaphragmatic Breathing

Deep breathing helps activate the parasympathetic nervous system, promoting relaxation and easing muscle tension. Sit upright, breathe deeply into your abdomen, and exhale slowly, focusing on steady, controlled breaths.

6. Seated Guided Meditation

Meditation can sharpen focus, reduce stress, and promote mental peace. While seated, close your eyes, focus on your breath or sensations, repeat a mantra or visualize an image, and calmly redirect your mind when it wanders.

These chair yoga exercises offer seniors an accessible and adaptable way to incorporate physical and mental wellness into their routine.

Chair Yoga Poses for Seniors

Yoga can be practiced conveniently, whether at home or in the office—even without leaving your desk! Below are some beginner-friendly chair yoga poses that seniors can easily incorporate into their routines. Remember to perform these poses slowly and gently, and feel free to use props for extra support if needed.

1. Seated Forward Bend
   - Sit at the edge of the chair with feet hip-width apart.
   - Inhale to lengthen your spine, then exhale and bend forward from the hips.
   - Rest your hands on your knees or reach toward the floor.
   - Hold for 5-7 breaths.

2. Seated Cat-Cow Stretch
   - With your feet flat on the floor and hands on your knees, inhale to arch your back and lift your chest (Cow Pose).
   - Exhale, rounding your spine and tucking your chin to your chest (Cat Pose).
   - Repeat for 5-7 breaths.

3. Seated Warrior
- Sit at the edge of the chair with your feet wide apart.
- Inhale, raising your arms overhead and clasping your hands together.
- Exhale and lean to the right, stretching your left side.
- Hold for a few breaths, then repeat on the other side.

4. Seated Eagle Arms
- Sit tall with your arms extended in front of you.
- Cross your right arm over your left, bringing your palms together.
- Bend your elbows, lifting your fingertips toward the ceiling.
- Hold for a few breaths, then switch the arm crossing.

Getting Started

Chair yoga is an excellent exercise for improving posture, enhancing flexibility, and boosting balance, all while minimizing the risk of injury. A comprehensive exercise routine should include flexibility and balance training, and chair yoga provides an ideal starting point. However, the mindful nature of yoga encourages you to focus on how your body feels during each movement, while maintaining deep, steady breathing to stay centered. It's essential to distinguish between discomfort and pain during practice. By moving gently and gradually increasing intensity over time, you can safely enhance your practice.

Chair Yoga Safety Guidelines
- Breathe: Inhaling and exhaling with each movement helps joints relax.
- Sit upright
- Align your knee over your ankle
- Keep your feet flat on the floor
- Avoid strain

- Refrain from jerking or bouncing movements

Breathing Techniques for Chair Yoga

If you've ever felt stressed or anxious, you've likely been told to take a deep breath. Although it may seem difficult at the moment, deep breathing is scientifically proven to calm the nervous system and reduce anxiety. Whether you're anticipating an event or winding down after a stressful day, breathing exercises offer an accessible and effective way to manage stress. Regular practice not only provides immediate relief but can also improve sleep quality and mindfulness, contributing to better mental health over time.

What is Yoga Breathing?

Yoga breathing involves more deliberate and controlled breaths than everyday breathing. The technique typically requires inhaling through the nose for a few seconds, followed by exhaling through the nose for an equal duration, with the mouth closed. This approach focuses energy (prana) and calms the nervous system, promoting relaxation. Here's a list of my favorite yoga breathing exercises for you to try. Practicing them in the morning, before bed, or anytime during the day (even in traffic!) can help reduce stress and bring a sense of calm.

- ❖ Deep Belly Breathing

This technique uses the diaphragm to maximize lung capacity, pushing air deeply into the belly. Start by lying down or sitting comfortably, placing one hand on your chest and the other below your rib cage. Slowly inhale through your nose for five counts, feeling your belly rise. Then, exhale through your mouth for five counts, noticing your belly relax.

❖ Box Breathing

Box breathing is a powerful method for calming the mind and managing anxiety. Inhale for four counts, hold your breath for four counts, exhale for four counts, and then hold again for four counts. Visualizing the four sides of a box with each breath can enhance focus and promote relaxation. Repeat four times.

❖ Alternate Nostril Breathing

This exercise promotes balance and calm, making it a great complement to meditation. Sit comfortably and exhale fully. Place your right thumb over your right nostril, inhaling through your left nostril for five counts. Then, close the left nostril and exhale through the right. Inhale through the right, then switch nostrils and exhale through the left. Continue alternating for several minutes.

❖ Breath Retention

Breath retention involves holding your breath for short periods, which aids relaxation. Sit with your back straight, inhale for five seconds, then hold your breath for 10 seconds. Exhale slowly through your mouth and take a few regular breaths before repeating.

❖ Lion's Breath

This fun and energetic breathing technique releases tension. Inhale deeply, open your eyes wide, and exhale forcefully through your mouth with a "haaaa" sound, sticking out your tongue as you release the air. Engage the muscles in your throat to enhance the effect.

❖ Breath of Fire

This technique involves gentle inhalation followed by forceful exhalation. It helps relieve stress, boost concentration, and promote mindfulness. Sit cross-legged, inhale through your nose for five counts, then exhale forcefully through your nose while engaging your abdominal muscles. Repeat this cycle 10 times quickly, maintaining even lengths for both inhalation and exhalation.

Achieving Proper Posture and Alignment in Chair Pose

Follow this step-by-step guide to ensure correct alignment and posture in Chair Pose.

1. Establish Your Foundation
Begin by aligning your body from the ground up. Position your feet either together or hip-width apart. Spread your toes widely and root firmly into the tripod base of your feet for stability.

2. Focus on Pelvis and Lower Back Alignment

With your foundation in place, shift your attention to the pelvis and lower back. Alignment varies depending on your natural spinal curvature.

- If you have a pronounced lumbar curve, gently tuck your pelvis to reduce it.
- For those with a flatter lumbar spine, allow your pelvis to tilt forward slightly to maintain a natural curve in the lower back.
- If your spine is naturally neutral, focus on maintaining that balance without forcing any adjustments.

3. Refine Your Chair Pose

Engage your legs by gently squeezing them toward your body's midline to build stability and heat in the inner thighs. Ground yourself by rooting into your feet while simultaneously lengthening your spine, as if reaching the crown of your head toward the sky.

- Activate your core by drawing your belly button toward your spine and engaging your waist. Bring your lower ribs toward your back body, creating a long, stable torso.
- Lift your collarbones and engage your arms as if they were pulling you upward. You can keep your arms shoulder-width apart or bring your hands to prayer position. Regardless of your arm placement, focus on energetically drawing them toward your body's center.

4. Create Length in Your Pose

Finally, focus on aligning the upper part of your body. Keep your neck and head in line with your spine, which might feel like a slight chin tuck. Avoid craning your neck forward or backward. Maintain a steady gaze either down the line of your nose or forward in front of you. And remember, smile and enjoy the strength and stability of your well-aligned Chair Pose!

The Importance of Chair Yoga Warm-Ups

Warming up before practicing chair yoga is essential for preventing injury and improving performance. It only takes a few minutes but can increase blood flow to the muscles by as much as 75%. Traditionally, yoga warm-ups, such as sun salutations or vinyasa flows, are used to prepare the body. "Vinyasa" refers to linking breath with movement. Starting your practice by syncing breath with motion helps center the mind and body, allowing for a smoother, more mindful flow. Warm-up sequences can be seen as moving meditations, bringing clarity and purpose to your day by aligning the mind with the body.

When to Do Chair Yoga Warm-Ups

While warm-ups are generally performed at the beginning of a yoga session, they can be beneficial at other times too. For instance, doing chair yoga warm-ups at the end of a workday can leave you feeling more centered and energized for your commute and evening. You can also incorporate them throughout the day, whether you're at the doctor's office, on an airplane, commuting, or simply winding down at home.

How to Practice Chair Yoga Warm-Ups

When warming up for chair yoga, your pace is flexible—move as slowly or as quickly as your body and breath guide you. The key is to maintain a synchronized flow between your breath and movements. Before beginning, eliminate distractions by silencing your phone and computer. Chair yoga warm-ups are similar to mat-based yoga warm-ups, except they are done seated. Common warm-up exercises include pelvic tilts, cat/cow stretches, dancing cat, sun salutation arm movements, forward bends, twists, and side stretches. These movements will prepare your body for the practice ahead while helping you focus and relax.

Seated Yoga Warm-Ups for an Engaging and Accessible Practice

While I personally enjoy starting a longer practice lying down, beginning from a seated position is a close second, particularly in the morning when lying down again right after getting out of bed might not feel ideal. This approach is especially helpful for morning practices or classes. In the early evening, when mental fatigue sets in, starting in a seated position can help maintain alertness. Varying your starting position also adds an element of mental engagement, making your practice more stimulating. Seated warm-ups are also beneficial for individuals who may find reclining positions difficult due to minor conditions like seasonal colds or more significant issues such as GERD or vertigo, which can worsen when lying down. This seated sequence I've outlined combines both dynamic movements and static poses, effectively warming up the spine, hips, and shoulders for a more active practice. It can even be a short, stand-alone session.

Since many of us spend much of our day sitting, sitting on the ground can sometimes be challenging. Ensuring the right support under your hips is crucial, especially if you have tightness in your legs, hips, or lower back. You can use a blanket, block, or bolster to maintain proper spinal alignment. If you're short on time, consider reducing the duration of the first pose, skipping the repetition of pose three, or omitting the static version of pose six.

Dynamic and Static Seated Warm-Up Sequence

Virasana (Hero Pose) – Any Variation (1 to 5 Minutes)
This is an excellent pose for centering yourself at the start of practice. If you find discomfort in your legs, knees, or hips, opt for Sukhasana (Easy Pose). Focus on maintaining a neutral arch in your lower back and take time to tune into your body and breath. Set an intention for your practice.

Seated Cat-Cow in Hero Pose (6 Rounds)
Gently move your spine and hips in sync with your breath by practicing Cat-Cow while seated in Hero Pose or Sukhasana. This helps mobilize the joints and prepare your body for deeper movements.

Arms Overhead Pose (Bound Hands) in Hero Pose (30-60 Seconds, Twice)

In this seated variation of Urdva Hastasana, interlace your fingers and stretch your arms overhead, activating your upper back, shoulders, and arms. After 30-60 seconds, switch the interlace of your fingers and repeat.

Dynamic-to-Static Easy Sitting Side Bend

This pose stretches your waist, ribcage, and arms. Start in Easy Pose with a dynamic version, alternating between side bends for several rounds. Then hold a static side bend for 30 seconds on each side.

Upward Plank Pose (Version 2, 30-60 Seconds)

A seated backbend, this pose helps open the chest and prepares your body for backbends or other seated poses.

Dynamic-to-Static Easy Sitting Twist

This twisting movement enhances spinal mobility and flexibility. Alternate between dynamic twists for several rounds, then hold each twist statically for 30-60 seconds on each side.

Easy Sitting Pose (Forward Bend, 30-60 Seconds, Twice)

This pose improves flexibility in the hips and spine. Practice with your shins crossed in front of each other, alternating sides after 30-60 seconds.

Boat Pose (Version 2, 30 Seconds, Twice)

A modified version of Boat Pose, this strengthens the core and leg muscles. It's a gentler variation for beginners or those recovering from illness. Hold the pose for 6-8 breaths and repeat if desired.

After completing the sequence, stretch your legs and transition to the rest of your practice.

Seated and Standing Chair Yoga Poses

Chair Yoga Seated Poses

Yoga, when practiced consistently, has been proven to enhance overall health. Like many exercise forms, it can be tailored to accommodate individuals of varying abilities. Chair yoga is a gentle form of yoga that can be performed either while seated in a chair or standing while using the chair for support. The benefits of chair yoga include:

- Improved flexibility
- Enhanced concentration
- Increased strength
- Improved mood
- Reduced stress and joint strain

Chair yoga can be done almost anywhere you can find a seat, making it accessible to those with limited mobility or for those looking to practice yoga while at work. Below are some foundational chair yoga poses to get you started:

1. Seated Cat-Cow Pose:
Begin by placing your hands on your thighs and sitting tall. As you exhale, round your back, pull your abdominals toward your spine, tuck your tailbone, and lower your chin to your chest—this is the Cat pose. On the inhale, arch your back, push your sternum forward, and lift your gaze (or keep your head parallel to the floor) for the Cow pose. Repeat this sequence, inhaling into Cow and exhaling into Cat, several times.

2. Seated Twist:
Place your left hand on your right knee and your right arm over the back of the chair. Turn your head to look over your right shoulder and hold for four breaths. With each inhale, lengthen your spine, and with each exhale, deepen the twist. Repeat on the other side.

3. Seated Chest Opener:
Sit at the edge of your chair and interlace your fingers behind your back. As you inhale, lift your hands up and away from your back while gently lifting your chin. As you exhale, release your hands. Repeat for a few breaths, then switch the grip of your hands and repeat.

4. Chair Pigeon/Hip Opener:

Place your right ankle over your left knee, allowing the right knee to relax outward while keeping the foot flexed. Sit tall as you inhale, and enjoy the stretch as you exhale. To deepen the stretch, gently press down on your right knee with your hand. For an even greater stretch, hinge forward from your hips while maintaining a flat back. Hold for three to five breaths, then switch sides.

5. Seated Forward Fold:

With your hands on your thighs, inhale deeply. As you exhale, hinge forward from the hips, draping your body over your legs. Let your hands slide toward the floor and either hold each elbow or let your arms dangle freely. Relax your head and neck, then slowly roll back up to sit on an inhale. Repeat several times.

6. Chair Downward Facing Dog:

Stand facing the chair, bend at the waist, and place your hands on the seat. Rotate your shoulders externally, pulling them away from your ears. Feel a stretch in your hamstrings and back. Hold for three breaths, then stand upright to release.

7. Chair Side Stretch:

Sit with your feet hip-width apart. As you inhale, extend your right arm up and over to the left side. For balance, place your left hand across your lap, holding your right leg or the chair. Breathe into your right side for three breaths, return to center, and repeat on the other side.

8. Chair Warrior II:

From a seated position, swing your left leg around the back of the chair, pressing your right foot down and grounding the outer edge of your left foot. Engage your core and lift your arms to shoulder height, looking over your right arm. Hold for three breaths, then switch sides.

9. Chair Reverse Warrior II:

From the Chair Warrior II position, slowly lift your right arm toward the ceiling while lowering your left hand to rest on your left calf. Feel the stretch along the front of your right side, holding for three breaths before switching sides.

10. Chair Eagle Pose:

While seated upright, cross your right thigh over your left, and if possible, wrap your right foot around your left calf. Cross your left arm over your right, bending at the elbows, and try to bring your palms together. Lift your elbows to shoulder height while pulling your shoulders away from your ears. Hold for three breaths, then repeat on the other side.

These chair yoga poses provide a convenient and effective way to improve flexibility, strength, and mental focus, making them ideal for individuals with limited mobility or those seeking a quick yoga practice throughout the day.

Standing Poses with Chair Support

1. Tree Pose:
This standing asana strengthens the legs and ankles while challenging balance. By incorporating the chair for support, the balance aspect is reduced, allowing participants to feel more grounded and focus on the hip-opening benefits of the pose.

2. Warrior III:
This pose challenges the hips and pelvis with legs placed in opposite directions. Using a chair removes the balancing difficulty, enabling a greater focus on pelvic stability. For individuals who have experienced falls, practicing this pose dynamically (transitioning from Mountain Pose to Warrior III with chair support) can be empowering.

3. Revolved Triangle:
In this pose, the leg muscles actively stabilize the body during the twist, making it challenging, especially with limited hamstring or abductor flexibility. Adapting the pose with a chair allows for greater emphasis on the twist while maintaining balance and proper spinal alignment.

4. Floating Half Moon:
This is a challenging balancing pose that requires openness in the front of the body to fully experience its benefits. Using a wall or chair for support enhances the sense of power, balance, and

alignment, enabling participants to experience the full effect of the pose with ease.

5. Chair Pose:

Often referred to as a squat, this pose strengthens the legs. However, for those with limited mobility, achieving the necessary depth can be difficult. Using a chair for support allows participants to feel secure while gradually progressing from a sit-to-stand motion to a low hover or squat. The positioning of the arms may vary depending on shoulder mobility, with "cactus arms" being a beneficial option for those with limited shoulder or latissimus dorsi strength.

6. Lunge:

This pose stretches the thighs, groin, and hip flexors while incorporating a gentle backbend. It requires balance and a degree of hip flexibility to maintain a long spine. The chair provides support, helping maintain balance and reducing the need to bend the spine forward, allowing participants to fully benefit from the pose.

Creating a Chair Yoga Routine

Looking to enhance your morning routine? Consider incorporating yoga into your start-of-day ritual. Yoga not only improves flexibility and strength but also boosts energy levels, alleviates stress and anxiety, and supports weight management. Regardless of your experience level, yoga offers benefits for everyone. Below are carefully curated routines designed for beginners, intermediates, and advanced practitioners to help you kickstart your day.

Beginner Routine

If you're new to yoga or prefer a gentle start, try this routine. Hold each of the five poses for 60 seconds before transitioning to the next. This should take about 5 minutes in total.

Child's Pose
An ideal way to begin your practice, especially in the morning, Child's Pose helps you reconnect with your breath while providing a gentle stretch for your lower back and hips.
Muscles Engaged: Lats, lower back, hips

Instructions:
- Begin on all fours on your mat.
- Spread your knees wide, with your big toes touching.
- Allow your stomach to fall between your thighs and rest your forehead on the floor.
- Extend your arms forward, palms facing down.
- Breathe deeply in this position.

Happy Baby

This pose directly stretches your lower back and hips.

Muscles Engaged: Hips, inner thighs, lower back

Instructions:
- Lie on your back on your mat.
- Bend your knees toward your stomach, grasping the outsides of your feet. Flex your heels and ankles.
- Maintain this position, focusing on keeping your ankles directly above your knees while gently pushing against your hands with your feet.

Cat-Cow

Warm up your body with Cat-Cow, which stretches the spine, engages the core, and opens the chest.

Muscles Engaged: Erector spinae, serratus anterior, abdominals

Instructions:
- Start on all fours with your hands under your shoulders and knees under your hips.

- Engage your abs, exhale, and arch your spine towards the ceiling, letting your head drop toward your chest. Hold for 10 seconds.
- Inhale and lower your spine, allowing your stomach to drop toward the ground as your head lifts. Hold for 10 seconds.

Cobra

Cobra Pose stretches the shoulders, chest, and abs, while also strengthening the arms and glutes.

Muscles Engaged: Lats, triceps, abdominals, glutes, hamstrings

Instructions:

- Lie on your stomach with your legs shoulder-width apart and the tops of your feet on the mat.
- Place your hands under your shoulders with elbows tucked in.
- Inhale and straighten your arms, pressing through the tops of your feet.
- Lift your chest off the floor and roll your shoulders back.
- Stop when your pelvis is no longer in contact with the ground and hold for up to 30 seconds.

Chair Pose

Chair Pose strengthens the legs, back, and shoulders while also challenging your balance.

Muscles Engaged: Abdominals, erector spinae, quads, hamstrings, gluteus medius, delts, triceps

Instructions:

- Stand with your feet together and inhale, extending your arms overhead.
- Exhale and begin to lower your hips, bending your knees until your thighs are parallel to the ground.
- Roll your shoulders down and back, pressing your tailbone toward the floor. Breathe deeply in this position.

Intermediate Routine

Elevate your practice with these six intermediate yoga poses, designed to enhance both flexibility and strength. Begin with a 2-3 minute warm-up using selected poses from the beginner routine if time permits. Hold each pose for 1 minute and complete the circuit twice for a comprehensive workout.

Downward Dog

A fundamental yoga pose that stretches the shoulders, hamstrings, calves, and feet while strengthening the arms and legs.

Muscles Worked: Quadriceps, Abdominals, Deltoids

Instructions:

- Start on all fours with your hands under your shoulders and knees under your hips.
- Inhale, then exhale and lift your knees off the ground, pushing your heels towards the floor and your tailbone up.
- Keep your shoulder blades drawn towards your tailbone and your head between your arms.
- Focus on grounding your feet.

Warrior I

This pose strengthens the legs and opens the hips and chest.

Muscles Worked: Abdominals, Hamstrings, Quadriceps

Instructions:

- Stand with feet together and arms at your sides.
- Step your left foot forward into a lunge, keeping the right leg straight and turning the right foot at a 45-degree angle.
- Extend your arms overhead, squeeze your shoulder blades down and together, and gaze upward at your fingertips.

Bridge

Enhance the strength of your posterior chain (the back of your body) with Bridge Pose.

Muscles Worked: Hamstrings, Glutes, Quadriceps

Instructions:

- Lie on your back with knees bent and feet flat on the ground. Place your arms at your sides, palms facing down.
- Inhale, then exhale and lift your hips towards the ceiling, pressing up through your feet.

Garland

This pose opens the hips, thighs, and ankles.

Muscles Worked: Deltoids, Abdominals

Instructions:

- Squat with feet close together and toes pointing out.
- Allow your torso to fall between your thighs, pressing your elbows against your knees.

- Keep your tailbone directed towards the ground and your chest lifted, using your knees for resistance.

Bow

Stretch the front of your body while strengthening your back with Bow Pose.

Muscles Worked: Lats, Triceps, Glutes, Hamstrings
Instructions:

- Lie on your stomach with arms extended by your sides and palms up.
- Bend your knees and reach back to grasp your ankles.
- Inhale, lift your heels away from your buttocks and your thighs off the ground, pressing your shoulder blades back and gazing forward.

Boat

Strengthen your core with Boat Pose.

Muscles Worked: Abdominals, Hip Flexors
Instructions:

- Sit with legs extended and lean back slightly, supporting yourself with your hands.
- Inhale and bring your knees towards your chest until your thighs are at a 45-degree angle to the ground.
- Extend your legs if possible, or keep them bent.
- Extend your arms parallel to the floor and hold.

This routine provides a balanced combination of stretching and strengthening exercises to help you build overall body strength and flexibility.

Advanced Routine

For experienced practitioners, this advanced sequence features seven poses designed to provide a comprehensive challenge. Begin with a warm-up from the beginner or intermediate routines, then proceed with this advanced circuit. Hold each pose for one minute and complete the sequence twice.

King Pigeon
This advanced variation of Pigeon Pose opens the hips and stretches the abdominals.
Muscles worked: Triceps, Biceps, Lats
Instructions:
- Start in Pigeon Pose with your left knee bent in front and right leg extended behind.
- Bend your right knee, bringing your foot towards your back.
- Arch your back and lower your head.
- Reach overhead to grasp your foot with both hands.

Dove
Dove Pose stretches the back and abdominals while strengthening the shoulders and legs.
Muscles worked: Deltoids, Quads, Hamstrings, Glutes

Instructions:
- Kneel on the floor with arms by your sides.
- Lean back onto your hands with fingers facing forward and arms straight.
- Lower onto your forearms.
- Push your thighs up and out, arch your back, and move your hands toward your feet.

Peacock

Peacock Pose develops arm strength and balance.

Muscles worked: Forearms, Abdominals, Lats, Low Back, Glutes, Hamstrings

Instructions:
- Kneel with wide knees and sit on your heels.
- Lean forward, placing palms on the floor with fingers pointing back.
- Bend elbows and position knees outside arms.
- Lean torso onto upper arms, lower head, then extend legs behind you.
- Shift weight forward and lift legs off the ground.

Lord of the Dance

This pose enhances balance, flexibility, and stretches the front of the body.

Muscles worked: Quads, Hamstrings, Abdominals, Lats

Instructions:
- Stand with feet together and arms by your sides.
- Bend your left knee, bringing your foot towards your butt.

- Grab the outside of your foot with your left hand, pushing your tailbone down and pelvis up.
- Extend your knee slightly upward, and extend your right arm forward parallel to the floor.

Headstand

Headstand builds upper body and core strength, improves balance, and enhances circulation.

Muscles worked: Triceps, Lats, Abdominals, Quads, Hamstrings

Instructions:

- Begin on all fours with wrists under shoulders and knees under hips.
- Place forearms on the floor, clasp hands, and position the top of your head in front of your hands.
- Straighten legs and walk them into a Downward Dog position.
- Lift one leg toward the ceiling, followed by the other.

Headstand Lotus

An advanced variation of the Headstand, this pose further challenges your balance.

Muscles worked: Triceps, Lats, Abdominals, Quads, Hamstrings

Instructions:

- Assume Headstand position.
- Bend your right leg and place it on your left thigh.
- Bend your left leg and position it on your right thigh.

Firefly

Firefly Pose stretches the hamstrings and hips while building arm strength.

Muscles worked: Deltoids, Lats, Triceps, Chest, Abdominals

Instructions:

- Squat and lean your torso forward between your legs.
- Place hands on the floor inside your legs, and bring upper arms close to upper thighs.
- Lift yourself off the ground, shifting weight into your hands, and extend legs forward.

Creating an ideal morning yoga routine, whether you're a novice or an advanced practitioner, can be a revitalizing and highly beneficial practice.

Chair Yoga for Specific Needs

Yoga for Joint Health

Yoga provides numerous health benefits, including enhanced flexibility, improved blood circulation, and accelerated injury recovery. It is also beneficial for joint health, which can become a concern with age. While all yoga poses contribute positively to your health, certain poses are particularly effective in promoting joint health and facilitating pain-free movement. Incorporate these poses if you're experiencing pain or focus on them proactively to strengthen your joints if you're not.

Bridge Pose
This pose is a variation of the bridge position often practiced in physical education or gymnastics. Lying on your yoga mat, bend your knees and place your feet flat on the floor. Gradually lift your body while keeping your head, neck, shoulders, and arms grounded on the mat. Ensure your thighs are parallel to the floor

and your knees are directly over your heels. The bridge pose strengthens the knee joints and is beneficial for individuals with osteoporosis.

Warrior Poses

The warrior sequence includes some of the most iconic yoga poses. Warrior I, II, and III involve standing with legs wide apart as if preparing for battle. With bent knees and elevated shoulders, these poses enhance balance and fortify knee joints. Warrior III, which requires lifting one leg to form a 90-degree angle, further strengthens the supporting knee and benefits the ankle joint.

Forward Fold

Recommended by the Johns Hopkins Arthritis Center, this pose is ideal for individuals with stiff muscles. It demands less flexibility compared to other poses and offers various adaptations based on your ability. Stand upright and fold forward at the hips, allowing your spine to roll forward until you are gazing at your shins. Bend your spine as much as possible, using a chair for support if needed. The forward fold strengthens the hips and knees while improving flexibility in the legs.

Plank Pose

This classic abdominal exercise is also excellent for joint health. Lying on your stomach, place your lower arms on the mat and bend your elbows at a 90-degree angle. Lift your body off the mat so that your weight is supported by your lower arms and toes. Aim to keep your body flat, which involves lowering your lower back and buttocks. The plank pose is a comprehensive strengthener, particularly beneficial for the wrists, arms, and legs. Aim to perform several sets, holding each for 30 seconds.

Bow Pose

The bow pose resembles a skydiving position on your yoga mat. Lying on your stomach, stretch your shoulders back and reach for your ankles with your arms. This pose is excellent for the shoulder joints and provides a significant stretch for your back and quadriceps.

Bound Angle Pose

Often included in cool-down exercises, this pose is also beneficial for the hip joint. Bend your knees and bring the soles of your feet together, tucking the heels as close to your pelvis as possible. Ideally, hold this pose for one to five minutes. It opens the hips and strengthens the knee joints.

Yoga Poses for Arthritis and Joint Pain

Is Yoga Beneficial for Arthritis?

Yoga is widely recognized as a beneficial practice for various types of arthritis. While arthritis varies in cause and symptoms, staying physically active is crucial alongside appropriate medical care. Research consistently supports yoga's efficacy in managing arthritis due to its ability to:

1. Offer Low-Impact Exercise: Yoga avoids high-impact movements like jumping, thus minimizing stress on the joints.

2. Be Inclusive: Yoga can be adapted for those with mobility issues. Many poses can be performed without leaving the mat, and chair yoga is a viable alternative. Studies show that individuals with lower body osteoarthritis experienced less pain and increased walking speed when participating in chair yoga compared to those in a health education program.

3. Alleviate Joint Stiffness and Pain: Yoga can significantly reduce stiffness and reliance on pain medication. Research indicates that individuals with knee osteoarthritis practicing yoga in conjunction with medical treatment reported decreased stiffness and pain compared to those receiving only medical care.

4. Enhance Muscle Strength: Stronger muscles support and reduce stress on the joints, improve balance, prevent bone loss, and lower fall risk. Individuals with lower body osteoarthritis face a significantly higher risk of falls, making muscle strength particularly important.

5. Improve Flexibility and Joint Mobility: Yoga increases flexibility and joint mobility, essential for daily functioning. A study found that just one week of yoga improved flexibility and range of motion in participants with knee osteoarthritis.

6. Boost Mental Health: Chronic pain and limited mobility associated with arthritis can contribute to depression and stress. Yoga has been shown to alleviate these symptoms, with studies noting reduced depression in individuals with rheumatoid or osteoarthritis after eight weeks of practice.

Recommended Yoga Poses for Arthritis

1. Low Cobra Pose: This gentle backbend enhances back strength and posture while stretching the chest and abdominal muscles.

Instructions:
- Lie face down on a yoga mat with legs extended and feet together. Place your palms under your shoulders and draw your elbows towards your body.
- Inhale, using your back muscles to lift your head and chest off the mat while keeping your neck long and shoulders away from your ears.
- Hold for 2-3 breaths, then lower your chest back to the ground. Repeat 5 times.

2. Chair Pose: Strengthens the muscles supporting the knee joint. For added stability, use a wall or start from a seated position.

Instructions:
- Stand with feet shoulder-width apart, engaging your core to support your spine.

- Exhale and bend your knees as if sitting in a chair, raising your arms overhead. Keep your spine straight and chest open, with most weight on your heels.
- Hold for 5 breaths, then inhale to extend your legs and lower your arms.
- For a seated variation, lift your buttocks an inch off the chair while holding your arms in front of you, then sit back down after 5 breaths.

3. Tree Pose: Improves balance and can be supported by a wall if needed.

Instructions:
- Stand with feet together, engage your core, and focus on a point in front of you.
- Shift weight to the right foot, lift the left foot and place it on the inside of your right calf or thigh (avoiding the knee).
- Extend through your torso and head, breathing deeply. Optionally, raise your arms overhead.
- Return to the starting position and repeat on the other side.

4. Cat-Cow Pose: Enhances mobility in the neck, shoulders, chest, and spine. Move slowly and synchronize with your breath.

Instructions:
- Begin on all fours with shoulders over wrists and hips over knees. Engage your core and maintain a neutral spine.

- Exhale, round your back toward the ceiling, and tuck your chin to your chest.
- Inhale, arch your back, drop your belly toward the mat, and look ahead or up.
- Alternate between these positions with your breath. For a chair variation, hold the seat edges and perform the movements seated.

5. Seated Spinal Twist: Increases spinal mobility and builds core strength.

Instructions:

- Sit on your mat with legs extended and spine straight, engaging your core.
- Bend your right knee, placing the foot outside your left hip.
- Inhale, reach your left arm up, then exhale and twist your torso to the right, placing your right hand behind you and keeping hips facing forward.
- Tuck your left elbow outside your right thigh and optionally press your forearm against your thigh for leverage.
- Hold for a few breaths, elongate your spine, and repeat on the other side.

Yoga for Back Pain Relief

Experiencing back pain is a common issue, often affecting the lower back (lumbago), though mid and upper back pain can also occur. Research indicates that yoga can serve as an effective complementary therapy for alleviating back pain, and many healthcare professionals endorse its use for this purpose. If you or someone you know is dealing with back pain and has been advised by a healthcare provider or physiotherapist to try yoga, selecting the appropriate poses is crucial. This section explores seven gentle yoga poses designed to help relieve back pain, offering guidance on how to approach these poses when dealing with an injury or during recovery. If experiencing severe or sharp back pain, consult with your doctor before beginning or continuing any yoga practice. Additionally, different types and causes of back pain may require different approaches; for instance, poses that alleviate lower back pain and sciatica might differ from those beneficial for upper back and neck pain. Always listen to your body and transition in and out of poses gradually to avoid exacerbating your pain. If uncertain, seek advice from a physical therapist or consider private yoga sessions for personalized feedback and adjustments.

Gentle Yoga Sequence for Back Pain

When starting yoga to manage back pain, begin with a slow and gentle practice, focusing on breathing. Begin with a short session of a few poses, observing how your back feels before, during, and after. If you experience reduced pain, this indicates that the practice is beneficial. Gradually extend the duration of your sessions as needed. The following seven poses can be performed together in a 15-minute routine or individually.

1. Child's Pose (Balasana): This pose allows the spine to gently round and stretches the back. It can alleviate discomfort from prolonged sitting. With knees slightly apart and big toes touching, sink your hips toward your heels, keeping your spine long and arms extended. Rest your forehead on the ground or a cushion for added comfort. Adjust knee placement to find what relieves your back pain best and focus on slow, deep breathing.

2. Cat-Cow Pose (Marjaryasana): This dynamic movement improves spinal flexibility and relieves tension. Start on all fours, with knees under hips and hands under shoulders. Inhale to arch your back and open your chest, then exhale to round your back and tuck your chin. Perform 3-5 slow rounds, syncing each movement with your breath.

3. Revolved Child's Pose (Parivritta Balasana): This pose introduces a gentle twist that can relieve back pain. From all fours, reach your right arm under your left and place your forearm

on the ground. Drop your right shoulder and ear, and extend your arm through to the left. To exit, press into your left hand and inhale to rise. Repeat on the left side.

4. Bound Angle Pose (Baddha Konasana): Hip tightness can contribute to back pain, so this pose helps open the hips. Sit with feet together and knees apart. Use a block or cushion if needed for support. Sit tall, lengthening your lower back, and if comfortable, lean slightly forward. Hold for 5-10 breaths, increasing time as comfort allows.

5. Seated Spinal Twist (Ardha Matsyandrasana): This twist improves spinal mobility. Sit with legs extended, bend the right knee, and place the foot over the left leg. Inhale to lengthen the spine and lift the left arm, then exhale to twist, placing the right fingertips behind you and hugging the left knee if needed. Hold for five deep breaths.

6. Knees-to-Chest Pose (Apanasana): This pose stretches and relaxes the spine. Lie on your back, hugging your knees to your chest. Gently rock or make small circles with your knees to massage the lower back. Continue with slow, deep breaths for 5-10 breaths.

7. Corpse Pose Variation (Savasana): This variation supports the lower back by keeping knees bent and feet apart. Lie on your back with knees bent and feet slightly wider than hips, allowing knees to touch without effort. Soften your abdomen and relax,

focusing on deep breathing. Stay in this position for 10 breaths to 10 minutes.

Yoga for Enhanced Circulation

Yoga has long been recognized for its health benefits, including its positive effects on circulation. Through various postures (asanas), yoga enhances blood flow by stretching, strengthening, twisting, and compressing the body. Combined with breathing techniques (pranayama), yoga can also help manage high blood pressure and improve circulation within the body's tissues. Regardless of the yoga style or method, regular practice can enhance your circulatory system. You do not need to be an advanced practitioner or exceptionally fit to benefit from yoga's circulatory improvements. Consistent weekly yoga sessions can significantly boost blood circulation and overall health.

1. Downward Facing Dog Pose: This pose promotes blood flow to the brain and upper body. By inverting the body into an "inverted V" shape with hands and feet on the floor, this posture enhances circulation to the head and neck. Keep your heels reaching toward the floor and your head between your arms. Maintain this position for several breaths.

2. Plow Pose: This pose aids in regulating digestion, strengthening the spine, and increasing blood flow to the thyroid gland. Lie on your back, extend your legs upward, and lower them slowly over your head. Support your lower back with your hands as you touch your toes to the floor behind you. After touching the floor, remove your hands from your back and hold this pose for 20-30 seconds while breathing comfortably.

3. Shoulder Stand Pose: This inversion reverses blood flow towards the heart and enhances circulation to the brain, also helping to alleviate fatigue and calm the mind. Lie on a folded blanket under your shoulder blades with your head on the floor. Lift your legs and hips vertically, balancing on your shoulders and upper arms. Support your back with your hands and hold this position for 5-10 breaths.

4. Standing Forward Fold Pose: This pose increases blood flow to the legs and feet and alleviates tension in the back and neck. Stand with feet hip-width apart, bend forward from the waist with knees slightly bent, and touch your hands to the floor. Ensure your back remains straight and your neck relaxed. Hold for 1-2 minutes, allowing your thighs and lower back to release tension.

5. Cobra Pose: This posture stimulates blood flow to the digestive organs, aiding in the relief of gas and bloating while stretching the back muscles and reducing stress. Lie on your stomach, extend your legs, and place your hands under your shoulders. Lift your chest off the mat while aligning your back and head. Hold this position for a few breaths before resting.

6. Warrior II Pose: This pose enhances circulation in the legs by strengthening and compressing muscle tissue and veins. From the back of your mat, step your right foot forward and align your left foot parallel to the mat. Bend your right knee to 90 degrees without letting it extend beyond your toes. Extend your arms to the sides and engage your legs. Hold for 5-6 breaths and repeat on the opposite side.

7. Legs-Up-The-Wall Pose: This pose helps drain excess blood from the lower extremities and alleviates stress and high blood pressure. Sit sideways on a folded blanket against a wall, lift your legs up against the wall, and lay back comfortably. Keep your legs fully extended and your arms spread out, palms facing up. Relax and breathe evenly while holding this pose for 5-8 minutes.

8. Seated Twist Pose: Begin seated with knees bent and feet near your left buttock. Inhale with a straight spine and lifted chest, then exhale while rotating your torso to the right. Place your right hand on the floor behind you and your left hand on your right knee. Continue to twist slightly more with each exhale and look over your right shoulder. Hold for 20-30 seconds, then switch sides.

Yoga for Improved Balance

For active older adults, maintaining good balance, gait, and range of motion is essential for overall health and well-being. As we age, there is a natural decline in muscle mass and metabolism, and sedentary seniors often face challenges with balance. However, active seniors who engage in balance training are typically better equipped to handle the demands of daily life and avoid falls. According to the Centers for Disease Control and Prevention, one-third of Americans over 65 will experience a fall each year. Falls are the second leading cause of brain and spinal cord injuries in older adults, making balance training crucial at this stage of life. Yoga is a highly effective method for improving balance, and for those unable to attend traditional yoga classes, many exercises can be performed with the support of a chair. Chair yoga incorporates flexibility and balance training, offering a sequence of static and dynamic poses to enhance daily living activities. Each pose should be practiced for about 30 seconds.

Gait Awareness

Focus: Enhances balance in motion and awareness of foot placement

How to Perform:

- Position a chair at one end of the yoga mat.
- Sit at the center of the chair with a neutral spine and feet flat on the floor.
- Concentrate on your foot placement on the mat.
- Place your hands on your thighs and rise to a standing position. Walk slowly to the opposite end of the mat, paying attention to how your heel, metatarsals, and toes make contact with the floor. Return to the chair, turn around, sit down, and repeat.

Progression: Walk backward toward the chair.

Downward Facing Dog

Focus: Enhances balance while in an inverted position (head below the hips)

How to Perform:

- Stand facing the chair's base.
- Inhale and raise your arms overhead.
- Exhale and place your hands on the chair's base (bending your knees if necessary).
- Gradually walk your feet backward and lift your hips until you achieve the down-dog position.
- To exit, walk your feet forward into a forward fold and roll up one vertebra at a time to stand.

Regression: Place your hands on the back of the chair.

Tree Pose

Focus: Develops single-leg balance

How to Perform:

- Stand next to the back of the chair with the chair on your right side.
- Place your right hand on the chair.
- Rotate your left leg outward, placing your left foot either above your ankle or on your calf.
- Raise your left arm overhead and hold.
- Repeat on the other side.

Progression: Release your grip on the chair.

Foot to Seat Pose

Focus: Develops single-leg balance and stepping motion

How to Perform:
- Stand facing the side of the chair.
- Place your left hand on the back of the chair and step your right foot onto the chair's seat.
- Keep your right hand on your hip or lift it overhead.
- Hold and then switch to the opposite side.

Regression: From a seated position, lift and hold one leg at 90 degrees.

Triangle Pose

Focus: Improves balance in a unilateral stance
How to Perform:
- Stand sideways next to a chair, with feet 3 to 4 feet apart.
- Turn the toes of the foot farthest from the chair 45 degrees and point the toes of the other foot toward the chair.
- Inhale and raise your arms to shoulder height.
- Exhale and reach the arm closest to the chair to rest on the seat or back of the chair, based on your flexibility.
- Hold and then repeat on the opposite side.

Progression: Look up toward the ceiling.

Palm Tree Pose

Focus: Enhances balance while standing on toes
How to Perform:
- Stand facing the back of the chair.
- Hold the chair's back and rise onto the balls of your feet.
- Lift one arm overhead, hold for several seconds, and then lift the opposite arm.

Regression: Lift one foot at a time while raising the opposing arm.

Moving Crescent Moon

Focus: Improves transitional balance

How to Perform:

- Stand behind the chair with both hands on its back.
- Reach the left hand upward, shifting your weight to the right leg while lifting your left heel off the floor, mimicking a side stretch.
- Return to center and place both hands on the chair.
- Reach the right arm upward, stretching toward the left, and lift the right heel off the floor.
- Continue alternating sides.

Regression: Perform this movement while seated in the chair.

Enhancing Your Practice Through Mindfulness and Meditation

Essential Elements of Mindfulness and Meditation Yoga for Seniors

1. Gentle Movement and Breath Awareness

Chair yoga focuses on slow, deliberate movements combined with breath awareness. This mindful approach helps seniors become attuned to their bodies, fostering a sense of calm and relaxation. The gentle nature of the practice allows participants to progress at their own pace, encouraging a non-judgmental and accepting attitude.

2. Seated Meditation Practices

Chair yoga integrates meditation practices, allowing seniors to center their attention on the present moment and develop mindfulness. Techniques such as guided visualization and body scans create a mental refuge, providing relief from daily stresses.

3. Social Connection

Yoga classes for seniors often function as social gatherings, fostering connections among participants. This shared experience builds a sense of community, reducing feelings of isolation and loneliness. The social benefits complement the physical and mental advantages of chair yoga.

How Mindfulness, Meditation, and Chair Yoga Can Enrich Seniors' Lives

1. Stress Reduction and Emotional Wellbeing
Mindfulness and meditation have been proven to alleviate stress and anxiety in seniors. By focusing on the present, individuals can better handle the challenges of aging, leading to enhanced emotional wellbeing.

2. Improved Cognitive Function
Mindfulness practices are associated with improved cognitive function. Seniors who engage in meditation may see enhancements in memory, attention, and overall cognitive abilities, leading to a sharper and more focused mind. This is particularly beneficial for residents in Memory Support Units and can help manage or prevent sundowning behaviors in individuals with Alzheimer's and dementia.

3. Enhanced Physical Health
The gentle movements and stretches of chair yoga improve physical health by increasing flexibility, joint mobility, and muscle strength. These benefits can positively affect daily activities, supporting independence and a higher quality of life.

4. Embracing Serenity
Integrating mindfulness, meditation, and chair yoga into seniors' lives offers a profound gift of wellbeing. With guidance from an experienced instructor, chair yoga blends physical and mental practices to create a balanced and serene existence. Each breath serves as a reminder of the beauty and grace found in the later stages of life.

Integrating Mindfulness into Chair Yoga Practice

As seniors transition into their later years, they often face significant physical and emotional changes. While retirement can offer newfound freedom, it may also present its own challenges. During this period of change, mindfulness and meditation become invaluable tools for fostering inner peace and calm. This section will examine the benefits of mindfulness and meditation for seniors, explore various techniques they can integrate into their daily routines, and discuss how these practices enhance overall well-being.

Understanding Mindfulness

Mindfulness, with roots in ancient contemplative practices, has recently gained recognition for its profound effects on mental and emotional health. At its essence, mindfulness is about being fully present in the moment, free from judgment. For seniors, this practice can be especially beneficial, helping them navigate the complexities of aging with increased resilience.

The Practice of Meditation

Meditation, a fundamental aspect of mindfulness, offers seniors a valuable means to explore deeper levels of self-awareness and tranquility. Various meditation techniques are available, each catering to different preferences and needs.

- Guided Meditation

  For those new to meditation, guided sessions can be particularly beneficial. These involve listening to a trained instructor or a recorded session that offers gentle guidance, helping seniors focus and relax.

- Mindful Breathing

  Mindful breathing is a simple yet effective technique where seniors pay attention to their breath. By sitting or lying comfortably and focusing on the sensations of inhalation and exhalation, they can promote relaxation and a sense of stability.

Integrating Mindfulness and Meditation into Daily Life

Incorporating mindfulness and meditation into daily routines doesn't require complex rituals or extensive time commitments. Seniors can easily integrate these practices into their everyday lives, making them both accessible and sustainable.

Morning Mindfulness Rituals
Beginning the day with a brief mindfulness session can set a positive tone. Seniors might engage in mindful breathing while enjoying their morning tea or coffee, fully experiencing the flavors and aromas. This simple practice creates a mindful anchor that can influence the rest of the day.

Mindful Movement
Physical activities such as tai chi or gentle yoga can facilitate mindfulness. By focusing on bodily sensations and the rhythm of their movements, seniors can enhance both their physical health and mindfulness.

Mindful Eating
Turning mealtime into a mindful experience allows seniors to deepen their connection with their food. Paying close attention to the colors, textures, and flavors of their meals, and savoring each

bite, can lead to a more fulfilling and nourishing dining experience.

Overcoming Challenges
Despite the benefits of mindfulness and meditation, seniors may face obstacles such as physical limitations, health issues, or skepticism. Overcoming these challenges requires flexibility and compassion.

Adapted Practices
For seniors with physical constraints, adapted mindfulness practices can be beneficial. Seated meditation, chair yoga, or customized mindfulness exercises can make these practices accessible and enjoyable for everyone.

Community Support

Participating in mindfulness and meditation within a supportive community can help reduce skepticism and boost motivation. Seniors can benefit from joining local classes, community groups, or online forums to share their experiences and learn from others.

Mindfulness and Meditation from a Christian Perspective

In the Christian context, mindfulness and meditation acquire a distinctive dimension by integrating ancient contemplative practices with spiritual devotion. While secular mindfulness often emphasizes being present without judgment, Christian mindfulness focuses on aligning one's thoughts and emotions with the divine. Christian meditation frequently involves reflecting on Scripture, contemplating the teachings of Jesus, and nurturing a deep connection with God through prayer. Instead of emptying the mind, Christian meditation aims to fill it with the Word of God and align it with divine purpose. This approach highlights the transformative power of faith and seeks to cultivate inner peace and calm through a profound spiritual connection, offering a sacred space for communion with God amidst life's challenges and joys.

Tips for Christian Meditation

Incorporating Christian meditation into your spiritual practice can be deeply enriching. Begin by selecting a quiet and comfortable space free from distractions. Choose a Bible verse or passage that resonates with you and spend time reflecting on its significance. As you assume a relaxed posture, close your eyes and breathe deeply, inviting the presence of the Holy Spirit. Silently repeat the chosen scripture, allowing its words to fill your heart and mind. Maintain a receptive posture, opening yourself to God's guidance and revelation. Consider using Christian music or hymns to enhance the meditative environment. Regular practice is important, so aim for a consistent routine that fits your schedule. Through these dedicated moments of Christian meditation, you can deepen your spiritual connection, foster inner peace, and experience the transformative impact of God's Word in your daily life.

Breathing Exercises

In yoga, breathing practices are known as pranayama, which translates to "breath control." These exercises are designed to harness the breath to benefit the practitioner. The term prana means "breath" or "vital energy" in Sanskrit, and ayama means "control." Thus, pranayama focuses on controlling the breath to influence both physical and mental states. Various pranayama techniques exist, including ujjayi, kapalabhati, kumbhaka, sitali, bhastrika, viloma, and alternate nostril breathing. These techniques are utilized in chair yoga as they would be in any yoga class.

The Power of Breath

Breathing is a crucial tool for altering our mental state. For instance, people often notice they hold their breath when stressed or take shallow, rapid breaths when hurried. Mastery of proper breathing can significantly enhance both mental and physical health, and improve overall well-being. Effective breathing also makes physical exercises more manageable, which is why it is integral to chair yoga practice.

Take a Deep Breath

Many of us have experienced someone advising us to "take a deep breath" during moments of distress. This simple act of deep breathing can be profoundly calming and transformative, shifting our emotional state and improving our sense of well-being.

In chair yoga, breathing exercises encourage us to focus on our breath, enhancing our awareness of life's vitality. Engaging in deep, slow breaths through the nose activates the parasympathetic nervous system, which helps to calm the body and increase oxygenation.

Benefits of Breathing Exercises for Chair Yoga
Each pranayama technique offers specific benefits:
- Ujjayi breathing helps to balance and calm the body.
- Kapalabhati cleanses the system.
- Kumbhaka (breath retention) enhances lung capacity.
- Alternate nostril breathing promotes relaxation.
- Bhastrika increases energy levels.
- Viloma teaches fuller breathing.
- Sitali cools and calms the body.

Relaxation Techniques

When traditional yoga practice—on a mat with various postures—may be impractical due to injury, limited mobility, or being confined to an office chair, chair yoga offers a viable alternative. This form of yoga allows you to experience the benefits of muscle and bone strengthening, balance, relaxation, and mind-body awareness while seated, whether at your desk or in your favorite chair at home. Chair yoga does not adhere to any single style but integrates and adapts poses from various yoga traditions. Even without extensive flexibility, participants can gain significant benefits from each posture. Ready to start? Try this brief sequence—just a few minutes long.

Begin by selecting a solid chair with a straight back. Start with a brief meditation to help calm your mind and prepare your body for relaxation. Sit comfortably with your spine straight and engage your core, grounding your tailbone into the chair. Inhale deeply, lifting your heart, and then exhale, relaxing your shoulders away from your ears. Inhale, reaching the crown of your head toward the ceiling. Close your eyes and focus on the point between your eyebrows, the center of will and spiritual perception. Continue to breathe slowly and deeply, allowing the world's concerns to dissipate and setting an intention for your practice.

1. Lotus Preparation (Padmasana): Traditionally used for meditation, the Lotus pose can be adapted to a desk chair. Sit upright with a straight neck and spine to calm your mind. Place your hands palms up with thumbs and first fingers touching. If possible, practice crossing your legs to approach the Lotus position, which can alleviate the stress of prolonged sitting. Perform the pose on both sides, practicing gently and listening to your body.

2. Eagle Arms (Garudasana): Sit up straight and extend your arms in front of you at a 90-degree angle. Cross your arms, placing the right arm over the left, interlock them, and press your palms together with fingers pointing upward. This pose strengthens the triceps, shoulders, and back muscles, and helps prevent carpal tunnel syndrome. For a similar stretch for the legs, cross and interlock them with one foot behind the other.

3. Knee Squeeze: Sit upright, inhale, and hug your left knee towards your chest, holding your breath momentarily. Exhale while lowering your head to your knee, holding for a few seconds while continuing to breathe deeply. Release slowly and repeat on the other side. This pose helps relax the lower back and supports digestion and respiration.

4. Mountain Pose (Tadasana): Adapt the traditional standing pose for sitting. Clasp your hands while inhaling, then exhale and extend your arms forward. Inhale again, turn your palms away from your body, and raise your arms until your palms face the ceiling. Stretch upward to feel taller. For a deeper stretch, bend your arms to each side. This pose alleviates stress in the head, neck, and shoulders, while lengthening the sides of your body.

5. Twist: Twists are beneficial for spinal health, strengthening abdominals and obliques, and detoxifying organs. Place your palms on the chair's armrests and inhale. Exhale, turning your chest and abdomen to the right, moving your left shoulder forward and right shoulder back. Imagine the twist beginning from the base of your spine. Inhale to expand your chest, and exhale to deepen the twist. Repeat on the other side.

6. Lunge (Anjaneyasana): Place your hands on the chair, inhale, and step your right foot onto the chair with your knee aligned over your ankle. Exhale, extending your left foot back into a low lunge. Hold for several breaths. This stretch benefits the hamstrings and strengthens the glutes and psoas muscles. Repeat on the other side.

7. Thread the Needle: Sit in your chair, cross your right leg over your left knee, and lift both feet off the floor. Clasp your hands around your left leg, just below the knee. This posture stretches the hip rotators and outer thighs, and relieves lower back tension. Be sure to switch sides.

8. Scale Pose: Place your palms on the chair's armrests and cross your legs at the ankles. Exhale, contract your abdominal muscles, and lift your buttocks and legs off the floor. Hold this position for five to eight breaths. Lower yourself, switch the cross of your legs, and repeat. If lifting yourself is challenging, start with lifting your buttocks and gradually add your feet as you build strength. This pose strengthens your arms, lower abs, and core.

9. Forward Fold (Uttanasana): Forward folds ease upper back and neck tension. Inhale deeply, then exhale as you bend forward, allowing your head and arms to hang heavily over your knees. Relax into the position, holding for several deep breaths. Inhale as you carefully return to a seated position.

10. Restorative Pose (Balasana): Restorative poses are essential for completing your practice. Clear your desk and inhale deeply. Cross your arms and place them on the surface in front of you. Exhale and rest your head on your crossed arms. This seated version of Child's Pose allows you to let go completely and breathe, finishing your practice with relaxation.

Adjust any of these poses as needed using breath and mind-body awareness. Consult your doctor before starting any new fitness routine, especially if you have health concerns, and avoid pushing your body beyond its limits. With a commitment to just five minutes of daily practice, you can enhance your flexibility, strength, and overall well-being.

The Importance of Rest and Recovery in Chair Yoga

The adage "less is more" can indeed apply to your yoga and fitness regimen. Although it may seem counterintuitive, incorporating rest days into your workout schedule is essential for:

- Enhancing stamina
- Improving muscle tone and repair
- Increasing flexibility
- Accelerating weight loss

Simply lounging on the couch isn't sufficient; a well-structured rest day plan is necessary to truly benefit from recovery. This chapter will clarify what constitutes a rest day, assess their suitability for you, and explain their importance. Additionally, we will differentiate between active and passive recovery and examine how yoga can serve as an effective method for active recovery.

What is a Rest Day?

A rest day involves taking a break from your regular exercise routine. It may involve minimal physical activity or an active recovery day where you engage in low-intensity exercises to support your body while still being active.

Active vs. Passive Rest Day Recovery

Different philosophies exist regarding rest days. It is essential to recognize that you know your body best and should trust your instincts to make the most appropriate choices.

What is Passive Recovery?

Passive recovery typically means complete rest from workouts. Activities on such a rest day might include:

- Reading
- Relaxing in a sauna
- Volunteering
- Spending time with loved ones
- Watching television

While these activities are beneficial, incorporating some active recovery is also recommended.

What is Active Recovery?

Active recovery involves engaging in low-intensity activities that keep your body moving while allowing muscles to recover. This approach helps stimulate cardiovascular function and circulation without overexerting your body. Effective methods for active recovery include:

- Gentle, restorative, or yin yoga
- Walking
- Cooling down after intense exercise (e.g., walking post-run)
- Swimming

Typically, active recovery is preferred over complete inactivity, though passive rest days are appropriate when you are exceptionally fatigued or burned out.

Who Should Take Rest Days?

Rest days are beneficial for everyone, regardless of whether you are new to exercise or a seasoned athlete. They are crucial for allowing your body to recuperate between workouts.

Why are Rest Days Important?

Rest days are vital for several reasons, including:

- Recovery and Repair: They allow muscles and tissues to heal, essential for maintaining fitness levels.
- Injury Prevention: Proper recovery helps prevent injuries, ensuring you can continue engaging in your preferred physical activities.

- Replenishment: Exercise depletes glycogen stores in muscles, and rest days help restore these energy reserves.
- Weight Loss and Muscle Building: Regular rest helps overcome plateaus in weight loss or muscle gain, preventing overtraining and enhancing adherence to long-term fitness goals.
- Mental Recovery: Physical activity can also strain the mind, and rest days support emotional and psychological well-being.

Signs You Might Need a Rest Day

Consider taking a rest day if you experience:
- Persistent muscle soreness and pain
- Quick burnout during workouts
- Mood disturbances such as insomnia or irritability
- A plateau in weight loss or muscle development

How Often Should I Take a Rest Day?

Typically, rest days are taken every 7-10 days. Adjust this frequency based on your personal fitness goals, the intensity of your activities, and your level of fitness. Beginners may require more frequent rest, while more experienced individuals might need fewer rest days.

Planned vs. Unplanned Rest Days

Maintaining consistency is crucial for achieving fitness goals. However, unplanned rest days can be necessary under certain conditions, such as:

- Illness: Avoid exercising if you're unwell to prevent worsening symptoms.
- Injury: Rest is essential if injured; focus on different muscle groups if possible.
- Exhaustion: If mentally or physically drained, listen to your body and prioritize rest to avoid injury and ensure proper form.

What to Do on a Rest Day

- To maximize rest days, consider:
- Hydration: Drink plenty of water to reduce muscle cramping and support recovery.
- Nutrition: Consume healthy carbohydrates to replenish glycogen levels, focusing on fruits and vegetables for optimal recovery.

Yoga for Active Recovery

Yoga is an excellent choice for active recovery. It is low-impact, requires only your body weight, and offers numerous styles to suit your needs. Practicing yoga on rest days enhances flexibility, breathing, circulation, and overall mind-body connection, helping to prevent burnout and maintain a balanced fitness routine.

Integrating Chair Yoga into Your Daily Routine

As we age, prioritizing physical well-being becomes essential. Chair yoga provides a gentle yet effective method for seniors to stay active, enhance flexibility, and cultivate a sense of calm. This step-by-step guide will help you seamlessly incorporate chair yoga into your daily routine, fostering a healthier and more balanced lifestylc.

Step 1: Establish a Consistent Schedule
Select a time each day that aligns with your schedule and energy levels. Whether in the morning to energize your day or in the evening for relaxation, maintaining consistency is crucial.

Step 2: Choose a Quiet and Comfortable Space
Identify a quiet area with ample room for your chair and arm movements. Ensure the space is free from clutter to create a serene environment for your practice.

Step 3: Invest in a Stable Chair
Opt for a sturdy chair without wheels that provides adequate support. Sit with your feet flat on the floor and maintain an upright, comfortable posture.

Step 4: Start with a Gentle Warm-Up
Begin your chair yoga session with gentle warm-up exercises. Rotate your ankles, wrists, and shoulders to increase blood flow and prepare your body for the poses ahead.

Step 5: Focus on Breath Awareness
Direct your attention to your breath. Inhale deeply through your nose, allowing your lungs to expand, and exhale slowly through your mouth. Conscious breathing fosters relaxation and improves concentration.

Step 6: Practice Seated Poses
Engage in a series of seated yoga poses, such as mountain poses, forward bends, and gentle twists. These poses improve flexibility and strength while minimizing joint strain.

Step 7: Include Arm Movements

Extend your arms in various directions with gentle movements to enhance upper body flexibility. This approach helps reduce tension and increases the range of motion.

Step 8: Embrace Mindfulness Meditation

Incorporate mindfulness meditation into your routine. Focus on the present moment, releasing stress and enhancing mental clarity. Utilize guided meditation or calming music as needed.

Step 9: Progress Gradually

As you gain confidence with chair yoga, gradually introduce new poses and movements. Listen to your body and avoid pushing beyond your comfort level.

Step 10: Cool Down and Relax

Conclude your chair yoga practice with a brief relaxation period. Sit comfortably, close your eyes, and focus on your breath. This step facilitates a smooth transition back to daily activities.

Incorporating chair yoga into your daily routine requires minimal time but offers significant physical and mental health benefits. By following this guide, seniors can enjoy the many advantages of chair yoga, enhancing overall well-being and vitality in their daily lives.

Practical Tips for Maintaining Consistency

Starting a yoga practice with enthusiasm only to let it lapse after a few days or weeks is a common experience, especially when life's demands take precedence. This is particularly true after disruptions like the festive season. However, getting back on track is manageable with the right approach.

Simplicity is key in resuming and maintaining your yoga routine. Yoga's essence lies in aligning the mind, body, and spirit, focusing on comfort and enjoyment rather than complexity or appearance. Sometimes, a brief stretch can help you reconnect and refocus. Here are some effective strategies for sustaining a consistent yoga practice:

1. Set Clear Goals
Reflect on your initial motivations for starting yoga, whether it's increased self-awareness, tranquility, or mindfulness. Identifying your purpose will help sustain your motivation.

2. Keep Your Practice Short and Simple
Consistent, brief sessions can be as effective as longer ones. Aim for shorter practices to prevent burnout and maintain motivation. Listen to your body's needs and adjust accordingly.

3. Adhere to a Schedule
Allocate a specific time each day for your yoga practice. Choose a time that fits your routine and stick to it to establish consistency.

4. Seek Inspiration and Motivation

Find a partner to hold you accountable, or share your goals with friends or family. Tracking your progress through photos or self-assessments can also keep you motivated.

5. Create a Dedicated Space

Designate a comfortable and inviting area in your home for yoga practice. Personalize this space with your favorite items to make it a pleasant environment.

6. Explore New Practices

Incorporate various yoga styles to keep your practice engaging. If you usually do vigorous yoga, try slower-paced styles like yin to create balance and prevent monotony.

7. Integrate Yoga into Daily Life

Yoga extends beyond asanas; it encompasses philosophical principles such as empathy, gratitude, and non-violence. Apply these values in your daily interactions to enhance your practice's impact.

8. Use Reminders

Place motivational reminders around your home to reinforce your goals. Display inspirational images, quotes, and milestones in frequently visited areas to keep your commitment in focus.

9. Reward Yourself

Positive reinforcement can boost consistency. Set rewards for meeting your practice goals, such as a spa day or new yoga gear. Treating yourself will encourage continued effort and dedication.

Integrating Yoga into Daily Activities

Modern life is often fast-paced, with our bodies, minds, and spirits constantly under stress. Balancing daily responsibilities can sometimes lead to neglecting our health and well-being. Yoga has long been valued for its ability to restore balance to the body, mind, and spirit, even for those with demanding schedules. The practice of yoga is flexible and can be incorporated into even the busiest of days with the right mindset. Here are five practical ways to integrate yoga into your routine, regardless of how hectic your schedule may be:

Start Your Day with Sun Salutations
The morning sets the tone for the day, and incorporating Sun Salutations into your routine can be highly beneficial. Aligning your wake-up time with the sunrise helps harmonize with the natural energy cycle. Aim for 6-8 hours of sleep and wake up around or before dawn. After your morning rituals, dedicate 10 minutes to Sun Salutations (Surya Namaskar), which can provide the benefits equivalent to a 40-45 minute workout, offering comprehensive mind-body-spirit health.

Practice Yogic Breathing Throughout the Day
Breathing is fundamental to life and directly affects overall health and wellness. Yoga teaches various pranayama techniques that can be performed anytime, anywhere. Full Yogic Breathing involves inhaling deeply, holding the breath for a few seconds, and exhaling slowly through the nostrils. This practice helps clear blockages in the body and mind while expelling toxins. Other techniques such as Alternate Nostril Breathing and Kapalbhati can also be beneficial.

Follow an Ayurvedic Diet
Ayurveda, the complementary science to yoga, plays a crucial role in sustaining a holistic lifestyle. The principles of Ayurveda focus on balancing the body's doshas, or constitutions, through diet. Adhering to a diet that suits your dosha can enhance the benefits of your yoga practice. Consult with an Ayurveda expert to determine your dosha and create a tailored dietary plan.

Incorporate Yoga Breaks
Even if you can't dedicate a specific time for yoga, short breaks throughout the day can be effective. Practice Chair Yoga poses such as Seated Spinal Twist, Cat/Cow Pose, and Seated Tree Pose during breaks at work, in the car, or at home. These simple, effective poses help maintain energy flow and support overall well-being.

End the Day with a 10-Minute Meditation
Before retiring for the night, spend a few minutes in meditation and self-reflection. Find a comfortable position and reflect on the positive aspects of your day with gratitude, while embracing any challenges with a positive outlook. This practice not only aids in better sleep but also brings peace to the mind and body.

Ultimately, embracing yoga begins with a resolution to integrate it into your life. With commitment and consistency, the practice will seamlessly fit into your daily routine.

Conclusion

Congratulations on Completing **Chair Yoga for Seniors Made Easy!** Whether you are new to chair yoga or have expanded your existing practice, I trust that this book has equipped you with valuable resources to enhance your well-being. You have learned how to practice chair yoga safely, explored poses suited to your body's needs, and discovered ways to incorporate mindfulness and relaxation into your daily routine.

As you continue on your chair yoga journey, remember that progress is the goal, not perfection. This practice encompasses not only physical movement but also the nurturing of your mind and spirit. Each stretch, breath, and moment of mindfulness brings you closer to a healthier and more balanced self. Listen to your body, celebrate small achievements, and take pride in every effort you make. Chair yoga is a versatile practice that can evolve with you, adapting to your needs over time. There is always something new to discover, whether it's refining a pose, deepening your breath, or simply finding more joy in the process. This journey is ongoing, offering continual opportunities for growth and well-being. I encourage you to maintain your practice. Even a few minutes of chair yoga each day can lead to significant improvements. Stay curious, stay committed, and, most importantly, be kind to yourself. The time and effort you invest in chair yoga are investments in your health, happiness, and overall quality of life.

Thank you for allowing me to be part of your journey.

.

.

Here's to many more days of gentle, fulfilling movement.

.

.

Keep breathing!
keep moving!!
and keep thriving!!!

I Have A Request

Thank You for Reading!

I sincerely hope you enjoyed Chair Yoga for Seniors Made Easy and found it helpful on your wellness journey. If this book brought value to your life, I kindly ask that you take a moment to leave a review on your preferred platform, whether it be on Amazon, Goodreads, or any other book review site. Your feedback is incredibly important and helps other readers discover the benefits of chair yoga. It would mean the world to me to hear your thoughts and experiences!

With gratitude,

Anne Herzog

HERE IS YOUR BONUS

DAY 1	Seated Mountain Pose (1 min)	Seated Forward Bend (1 min)	Seated Cat-Cow (5 rounds)	Seated Side Bend (30 seconds each side)	Seated Spinal Twist (1 min each side)	Seated Neck Stretches (30 seconds each side)
DAY 2	Seated Mountain Pose (1 min)	Seated Arm Circles (1 min)	Seated Warrior I (1 min each side)	Seated Warrior II (1 min each side)	Seated Leg Lifts (1 min each side)	Seated Ankle Rolls (30 seconds each side)
DAY 3	Seated Mountain Pose (1 min)	Seated Forward Bend (1 min)	Seated Tree Pose (1 min each side)	Seated Chair Pose (1 min)	Seated Shoulder Rolls (30 seconds)	Seated Spinal Twist (1 min each side)

DAY 4	Seated Mountain Pose (1 min)	Seated Deep Breathing (2 mins)	Seated Shoulder Rolls (30 seconds)	Seated Forward Bend (1 min)	Seated Eagle Arms (1 min)	Gentle Neck Stretches (30 seconds each side)
DAY 5	Seated Mountain Pose (1 min)	Seated Leg Lifts (1 min each leg)	Seated Boat Pose (1 min	Seated Forward Bend (1 min)	Seated Side Bends (30 seconds each side	Seated Spinal Twist (1 min each side)
DAY 6	Seated Mountain Pose (1 min)	Seated Forward Bend (1 min)	Seated Warrior I (1 min each side)	Seated Warrior II (1 min each side)	Seated Tree Pose (1 min each side)	Seated Ankle Rolls (30 seconds each side)
DAY 7	Seated Mountain Pose (1 min)	Seated Cat-Cow (5 rounds)	Seated Forward Bend (1 min)	Seated Shoulder Rolls (30 seconds)	Seated Spinal Twist (1 min each side)	Seated Deep Breathing with Guided Relaxation (5 mins)

DAY 8	Seated Mountain Pose (1 min)	Seated Forward Bend (1 min)	Seated Cat-Cow (5 rounds)	Seated Side Bend (30 seconds each side)	Seated Spinal Twist (1 min each side)	Seated Neck Stretches (30 seconds each side)
DAY 9	Seated Mountain Pose (1 min)	Seated Arm Circles (1 min)	Seated Warrior I (1 min each side)	Seated Warrior II (1 min each side)	Seated Leg Lifts (1 min each side)	Seated Ankle Rolls (30 seconds each side)
DAY 10	Seated Mountain Pose (1 min)	Seated Forward Bend (1 min)	Seated Tree Pose (1 min each side)	Seated Chair Pose (1 min)	Seated Shoulder Rolls (30 seconds)	Seated Spinal Twist (1 min each side)
DAY 11	Seated Mountain Pose (1 min)	Seated Deep Breathing (2 mins)	Seated Shoulder Rolls (30 seconds)	Seated Forward Bend (1 min)	Seated Eagle Arms (1 min)	Gentle Neck Stretches (30 seconds each side)
DAY 12	Seated	Seated	Seated	Seated	Seated	Seated

	Mountain Pose (1 min)	Leg Lifts (1 min each leg)	Boat Pose (1 min)	Forward Bend (1 min)	Side Bends (30 seconds each side)	Spinal Twist (1 min each side)
DAY 13	Seated Mountain Pose (1 min)	Seated Forward Bend (1 min)	Seated Warrior I (1 min each side)	Seated Warrior II (1 min each side)	Seated Tree Pose (1 min each side)	Seated Ankle Rolls (30 seconds each side)
DAY 14	Seated Mountain Pose (1 min)	Seated Cat-Cow (5 rounds)	Seated Forward Bend (1 min)	Seated Shoulder Rolls (30 seconds)	Seated Spinal Twist (1 min each side)	Seated Deep Breathing with Guided Relaxation (5 mins)